A true story about my approach to a deadly cancer.

How I Beat Pancreatic Cancer

And other bedtime stories!

How I Beat Pancreatic Cancer: And Other Bedtime Stories

© 2018 Robert Miller

ISBN-13: 978-1-946702-20-3

Freeze Time Media

A true story about my approach to a deadly cancer.

How I Beat

Pancreatic

Cancer

And other bedtime stories!

Robert Miller

Dedication

This book is dedicated to my wife, Diane, and my two sons, Christopher and Justin, who stood by me during the darkest days, and to the hundreds of thousands of famous and not so famous people who have been affected by this terrible cancer:

Aretha Franklin

Steve Jobs

Patrick Swayze

Alan Rickman

Jack Benny

Luciano Pavarotti

Joan Crawford

Sally Ride

Donna Reed

Marcello Mastroianni

John Hurt

Anne Francis

Count Basie

Pete Postlethwaite

Fred Gwynne

Ben Gazzara

Michael Landon

Rex Harrison

Alan Bates

Henry Mancini

Keenan Wynn

Melvin Belli

Fernando Lamas

Wernher von Braun

Pernell Roberts

Richard Crenna

Michael Deaver

William Safire

Simone Signoret

Dizzy Gillespie

Margaret Mead

Don Hewitt

M. Scott Peck

Fiorello H. LaGuardia

Lorraine Hansberry
Mickey Spillane
Mark Goodson
Madeline Carroll
Rene Magritte
Lily Pons
Juliet Prowse
Melvin Simon
Peggy Ann Garner
Gene Upshaw
Randy Pausch
George Halas
Frank Herbert
Vince Edwards
Harry Nilsson
Kenneth Mars
Roger Williams
Harve Presnell
Dith Pran
Chuck Daly
Griffin Bell
Irving Wallace
Charles Guggenheim
Frank Church
Joseph Cardinal Bernardin
Lillian Gordy Carter
Sam Rayburn

Tom Mankiewicz
Julius Carry
Denis Thatcher
Daniel Taradash
Richard Dean
David Loxton
Jerry Juhl
William Hootkins
James Earl Carter, Sr.
Charles Arnt
Axel Madsen
Danny Aiello III
L. Patrick Gray
Gareth Hunt
Vivien Thomas
Symona Boniface
Barbara Orbison
Hank Cochran
Emily Couric
Dorothy Arnold
Billy Carter
Winthrop Rockefeller
Webb Price
Patty Costello
Eddie Foy, Jr.
Jimmy Hanley
Sam DeLuca
Robert Joffe

Art Fleming
Tony Ryan
Oona O'Neill
Steve James
Wilye White
Paul Mitchell
Tex Williams
Ralph Bates
Kim Weiskopf
Diana Lewis
Michael J. Daly
Patrick Dennis
Terry O'Sullivan
Mike Dora
Christie Allen
John Sylvester White
Irving Stone
Carole C. Noon
Henry Burkhardt III
Roger Crozier
Ruth Carter Stapleton
Robert L. Howard
Jim Baxter
Sandy Scott
Vince McMahon, Sr.
Eden Ross Lipson
Gloria Carter Spann
Tony Mazzocchi

Colt Terry
Stephen L. Price
Robert Willis
Jay Schulberg
Suzanne Wright

Contents

1

I'M NOT FEELING VERY GOOD

I'm very much average. My entire life has been spent in the middle of the road. Most of us don't want to admit that we are average, but unfortunately, too often, that is the truth. With me being one of the masses, and just average, you probably want to know how I was able to beat pancreatic cancer. Was it the fact that I was treated with radiation, surgery, and chemotherapy that I survived? Perhaps! However, I seriously doubt my experience with the standard three regimens offered as a pancreatic cancer cure at the time was the only reason that I survived my maladies. When I was diagnosed (1996), the two-year survival rate for pancreatic cancer was less than five percent. The five-year survival rate was less than one percent (these statistics haven't changed much in the last twenty years).

The reason I have survived, and I say this with confidence, is because when I reached my fifth-year survival anniversary, I specifically asked each of my doctors if they would take credit for my being alive? The answer I received was a resounding "NO"! Each doctor did tell me they would love to take credit for my unusual results but in all honesty, they couldn't. However, the one thing that each one of them did tell me was, "Whatever you are doing...don't stop." Being a good patient, I took their advice! I have never stopped my *regimen* I began at the very beginning of my cancer treatments. That *regimen* came about after I read several books about cancer (all kinds of cancer and not just pancreatic cancer) and incorporating a lot of common sense. My cancer *regimen* is the subject of this book.

I'm not sure when my cancer developed, but I'm positive it was over a period of time (it has been estimated that it takes cancer at least ten years to grown into a one-centimeter mass). I know I gave the cancer all the necessary tools to manifest itself because of my lifestyle. I ate all of the wrong foods — a lot of meat, anything fried — and I was a very heavy drinker. I found myself to be forty-plus pounds overweight with combined cholesterol levels around three hundred forty.

My triglycerides were even higher. My family doctor put me on Lipitor in order to reduce my cholesterol. I took Lipitor, a statin drug, for just two weeks before I realized I was seriously ill with a lot more than high cholesterol.

2

AUGUST 1996

Diane, my wife, and I decided to go to one of our favorite Mexican restaurants for dinner as it was close to my birthday (August 19). I already had several vodka drinks and was feeling very good as I did most nights. You see, I was very happy in my marriage, had two terrific sons, two loving dogs, a very good group of friends, and a terrific job with no money worries. The job was a little stressful at times but nothing I couldn't handle. I was living the "*good life.*" My doctor had identified my cholesterol problem and given me the medicine that would correct it so I didn't have to change anything. I could keep living my life as I always had and everything would be all right. That's what I was led to believe.

All too often we want to go to the doctor and have them give us a pill to address our symptoms instead of finding the problems that are causing the symptoms. This is when we place false trust in our doctors and allow them to take control of our lives because we think they know what is best for our health and well-being. Nothing could be further from the truth. Had my doctor been really interested in my health and well-being he would have put me on a diet to reduce my cholesterol instead of prescribing Lipitor.

There is so much false information circulated in the general public about the benefits of various drugs it is hard to comprehend let alone understand. We assume because a drug has been approved by the FDA it must be safe. The FDA is not your friend. Seventy percent[1] of the FDA's budget comes from the drug companies, with some members of the FDA approval boards also being paid by the drug companies. Just keep in mind the FDA approved VIOXX manufactured by Merck Corporation. This medication was for arthritis and a painkiller. The medication hit the market in 1999. It was pulled in 2004 after one hundred fifty thousand people taking the drug had heart attacks and sixty thousand died. To date, Merck has paid seven billion dollars in settlements and fines. This is just one of the many cases of fraud

---

1   David Hilzenrath, 12/01/2016, POGO, www.POGO.org/our-work/reports/2016/FDA-depends-on-industry-funding.html

and bogus clinical studies approved by the FDA and their drug company staffs.

After a terrific dinner that involved some fried food, a lot of meat and at least four beers, plus the vodkas I had consumed earlier, we returned home. It was late so we went straight to bed. We had a high king size bed that I propped my rear end against as I bent over to remove my socks. Diane was in the bathroom and didn't hear me groan as I felt the horrific pain shoot through my chest just below my sternum. The pain was so great I imagined it must be similar to what it would feel like if you were stabbed in the chest with a long knife. The pain went from the front of my chest to my backbone. My only thought was I was having a heart attack. I sat up immediately and took a deep breath. The pain stopped. Everything seemed normal again. Needless to say, every possible thing I could imagine, given my limited knowledge of health issues, ran through my mind: heart attack, massive indigestion, reaction to the Lipitor, anything and everything — but nothing to do with cancer.

I was able to get into the bathroom and get myself ready for bed. I didn't say anything to Diane for fear of her worrying all night. Surprisingly, I was able to sleep despite the incident. I figured it was something to do with all the food I had consumed that evening. I didn't worry about it. It was probably something minor and likely not to return. I decided no more Mexican food late at night!

The next morning when I visited the bathroom to relieve myself, I was shocked to notice my urine was a bright orange color. At this point I started to really get concerned. The first thing I thought I was flirting with was some sort of liver cirrhosis. There wasn't any unusual pain except for the incident last night. I figured I should probably call my family physician. I did make the call, which was highly unusual for me to even consider going to the doctor. This was Thursday morning and the first appointment he had available was the following Tuesday.

Once I was in the doctor's office, he noticed the whites of my eyes were beginning to turn yellow, a sign of jaundice. He asked me if I ate raw fish (sushi), which I did. He asked me if I had access to well water, which I did. (We normally spent our weekends in the North Georgia Mountains at our cabin on Lake Burton. All the homes at the lake were on well water). Based on the fact I was jaundice, ate raw fish and drank well water, he immediately believed I had acquired hepatitis C.

He decided to run a blood test. The results would not be back for a week.

A week later the blood test results came back, and the hepatitis C findings were negative. My doctor was not convinced so he decided to rerun the test. He told me the test was not perfect and often offered a false positive/negative result. In other words, he told me, sometimes the tests results were right and sometimes they were wrong. It had now been two plus weeks since my episode after the Mexican food upload. I was becoming a deep yellow all over my body and the white of my eyes no longer existed — they were one hundred percent yellow. During this time period I had developed an itch all over my body. Nothing could quell the itching. I tried everything but nothing worked. I was miserable. I began to lose my appetite and started to lose weight.

My doctor was trying to prove to himself that I had hepatitis C, which certainly involved my liver. I had concerns of my own since I consumed a lot of alcohol. What would the final outcome be: hepatitis, cirrhosis or worse? I wasn't going to wait on the doctor and his tests that were "correct some of the time and were wrong some of the time." I started to think about what all this meant, then common sense kicked in and my options were clear! I immediately decided on the first step in my treatment protocol, though I didn't know it at the time: I had my last drink. That day, I stopped drinking alcohol of any kind. I can honestly say that I haven't had a drink from that day forward and it has now been more than twenty-one years!

After my doctor received the same results from the second hepatitis C test, he realized more testing was needed. Even though the preliminary focus was my liver, my doctor sent me to a gastrointestinal specialist who conducted an endoscopic test, which led to a sonogram. I was advised that they wanted to admit me to the hospital for further tests. I agreed and thus began the real search for my problem. After a couple of days of x-rays, blood test and more x-rays, my doctor introduced me to two new doctors: a surgeon and an oncologist. The surgeon explained to me that I had *pancreatic cancer*. I had no idea what that was? The only thing I heard was "cancer." My life was about to change forever.

The surgeon explained his part was to cut out the tumor. The oncologist would treat me with chemotherapy after the surgery to make sure I was cancer free. They told me that I would also need radiation but the radiologist wasn't able to attend the meeting at that time. They also explained that the type of cancer I had was very bad and it would be very difficult to realize a positive result. They assured me they were going to "try." I emphasis the word "try" as there was no discussion of a cure.

We discussed the options, which were limited. My best chance for any additional life was to have a Whipple procedure, which is a type of surgery, radiation and lots of chemotherapy.

The Whipple procedure is a type of surgery that was developed in the 1930s. Several doctors contributed to the development of this procedure over a forty-plus-year period, but Dr. Allen Oldfather Whipple ended up providing the best technique that is followed today. The discovery of vitamin K in the 1940s was also a major factor in the Whipple procedure being successful. Dr. Whipple performed thirty-seven of these procedures in his lifetime. The procedure generally lasts five to six hours.

I specifically asked the surgeon, "What is the survival rate for this serious operation?" His answer was, "The mortality rate is eighty percent." Not being very familiar with the term "mortality rate" and having requested the "survival rate,"

I immediately thought the survival rate was eighty percent. The odds sounded good to me so I said "OK!" Actually, only twenty percent of the surgery candidates at that time (1996) survived the operation. This procedure is a very serious and difficult operation. When the doctors left my room, nobody was smiling.

I now knew my problem — *I had pancreatic cancer!* Approximately twenty-five thousand men and women were diagnosed in 1996 with this terrible cancer. The survival rate for two years was around five percent. A five-year survival rate was extremely rare with only one percent living that long. Today there are fifty-five thousand plus new cases diagnosed with pancreatic cancer.[2] Pancreatic cancer has passed breast cancer as the third leading cause of cancer deaths in the United States. The death rate for pancreatic cancer has remained virtually unchanged in the last forty years.[3]

---

2   American Cancer Society estimate for 2018

3   CodePurpleNow. Suzanne Wright Foundation

3

SEPTEMBER 24, 1996

The doctors allowed me to return home for the weekend. I was to return to the hospital on Monday to prepare for my surgery on Tuesday, September 24. Before I left the hospital, the doctors inserted a stainless steel drain pipe into the lower lobe of my liver. This was done without any pain medication, as I had to be alert to move my body as instructed by the technician. He used x-ray equipment to insert the metal tube between my ribs and into the lower liver lobe. "OUCH" is all I can say about that. The drain protruded about three inches out from my back, with about two feet of plastic tubing attached to the exposed end. The idea was to drain bile from my liver that had been backing up because of the bile duct passing through my pancreas was closed by the tumor. Using gravity to create the flow, my new drain system worked quite well. Diane was to collect all the bile discharge, measure it and record the amount of liquid being drained. Over the weekend she collected five bags of liquid. The bags were similar in size to the plastic bags you see hanging in the hospital next to a patient's bed to administer a drip solution of saline. Even though the bile liquid was a brownish green, like the color of a rotting avocado that has been exposed to the air too long, much to our surprise, it didn't have any odor.

I arrived at the hospital at 7 a.m. Monday morning and checked myself in. I spent the morning going through a battery of tests and additional x-rays. Tuesday morning they moved me into the operating room. Six hours later, the doctors announced to Diane I had survived the operation ... it was a success and everything went well (I had not joined the eighty percent who didn't survive this operation). Next, we had to wait for the pathology report.

The surgeon met with Diane several hours later to inform her that the outcome of the operation wasn't as good as he had hoped. During the surgery, he had removed a 3cm adenocarcinoma tumor from the head of my pancreas, my gallbladder, one-fourth of my stomach, one-third of my pancreas, my duodenum and common bile duct. He also removed twelve lymph nodes in the pro-

cess. Of the twelve lymph nodes, two were positive for cancer. The cancer had metastasized.
It had entered my lymph system. At this point,
the doctors knew if I lived for a year I would be
extremely lucky. Later, when he met with Diane
and me, he suggested I should get my affairs in
order and hope for the best. This was his polite
way of saying, "You are going to die!"

I stayed in the hospital recovering for ten days
after the operation. My stay was uneventful except for the fact that a couple of nights after
my surgery I flat-lined ... *my heart stopped*! It ap-
peared that I had not been given any electrolytes
before and after the surgery. The heart will not
function without potassium, magnesium, sodium and calcium in your system. I'm not sure
if just one was low or all of them, but I officially
checked out. At this point, you can say whatever you want about hospital food and I will tend
to agree with you. Please keep in mind this was
1996 and nutrition was something that was associated with tree-huggers, long-haired hippies
and anti-government malcontents. Nutrition
was not on the menu (no pun intended) of the
medical establishment. Food was food and nothing more. In 1996, when a doctor told you what to
eat, it was normally "eat a low-fat *healthy* diet"...

what the hell is that? Unfortunately, today it is pretty much the same prescription — most doctors know nothing about a healthy diet!

Now, this event was an extremely important motivator in my thought process once I began to set up my regimen to fight my cancer. I was in a modern hospital, being attended to by excellent, well-educated physicians with all the latest equipment, yet I almost died after surviving a serious six-hour surgery. This really makes one question what was going on in the ICU. Where were all the well-trained technicians and doctors? The only reason for my close call with death was the lack of important minerals: potassium, magnesium, sodium and calcium (electrolytes) in my system! Hard to believe but, sadly, it was true.

In the July 26, 2000 issue of JAMA (Journal of the American Medical Association), a report documented over two hundred twenty-five thousand deaths each year due to medical errors. A similar study by Harvard University found over one million patients are injured by errors during hospital treatments annually, with over one hundred twenty thousand deaths. Fortunately, I didn't add to those numbers. Today, the estimate has been quoted as high as seven hundred fifty thousand deaths due to medical and hospital errors.

Actually, medical errors are the third leading cause of death behind heart disease and cancer in the U.S. "If heart disease or cancer doesn't kill you there is a good chance the health care system could."[4]

I had a really interesting experience when I regained consciousness after being moved from the ICU to my hospital room. When I opened my eyes and my mind began to clear from the anesthesia and all the pills I had been given, I immediately noticed a very large person sitting in the corner of the room. He had a Bible and seemed to be praying. As reality came rushing back to me, I realized it was my old friend Tom Allison, whom I hadn't seen since high school, thirty-five years earlier.

Tom Allison, the very first person I see after my life-threatening surgery and brief encounter with death, had been convicted of killing his parents. Tom had spent twenty-five years in prison as a guest of the State of Georgia. His story was the subject of a book by Ann Rule, an American crime author, who wrote about Tom's case in "Everything She Ever Wanted," which was made into a TV movie. While in prison, Tom began a ministry dedicated to helping other prisoners.

---

4   Theresa Sabo, Patients for Patient Safety Canada

When he was released, he set up a halfway house to continue that ministry and help ex-convicts adjust to life outside prison walls. Knowing Tom Allison's story, and Tom being the first person I set my eyes on after being in and out of consciousness for hours, still rather unclear in my thinking, quickly made me question if I had died? Was I in Heaven or was I in Hell?

After ten days in the hospital, I was released. I returned home to recuperate and prepare for my chemotherapy and radiation treatments, which would start approximately one month after my discharge. While recovering, I tried to read all the information I could about pancreatic cancer. The articles and material I read were not encouraging. They basically told me I was going to die. However, Lori Roberts, a good friend of Diane's, came to see me within a week of my returning home. She believed in homeopathic medicine. She brought me a book on cancer, "Beating Cancer with Nutrition," written by Dr. Patrick Quillin. I can honestly say it was the best gift I have ever received. It probably saved my life!

I began to read the book and found it very easy to understand and uplifting. I realized how much sense it made, especially his very direct statements regarding the current state of cancer treatment today. He wrote something that will remain with me forever. After reading his book, I was not able to get the following thought out of my mind. I'm paraphrasing here, but the thought goes something like this:

"Imagine a tree in the middle of the forest. It has mold growing on one side of it. You can cut the mold off. You can burn the mold off. You can spray chemicals on the mold to kill it. All of these things will remove the mold, but if you don't change the tree's environment, the mold will grow back"!

Whoa, that really made sense! I had spent my entire life eating badly and neglecting my nutrition; I knew then and there I needed to change everything about my lifestyle and diet. *Remember, the definition of an IDIOT is someone who does the same thing over and over expecting a different result.*

All of a sudden I had a road map to deal with my cancer. I didn't have to lie in bed and feel sorry for myself. I could join my doctors in the cancer battle and actually do something to help. I decided to change my lifestyle ... forever! No more stress. No more alcohol, which I had already stopped. No more beef. No more pork. No more hydrogenated oils. No more fried foods. As a part of being alive, you have to eat. Eating to help strengthen my immune system was now my first order of business. I could do this! Bring it on.

I had already committed to surgery, chemo and radiation for my treatment. Now, thanks to Dr. Quillin's book, I was bringing nutrition and supplements into the mix, things that would be considered "alternative cancer treatments," and things doctors wouldn't necessarily recognize as important. I decided to do both treatments, standard cancer treatment along with my new-found alternative approach, *simultaneously*, and here's why: In the early 1960s, I remember reading several of Kahlil Gibran's books, especially "The Prophet." In one of them he said, and again I paraphrase, *"There are so many roads to God, why limit yourself to just one?"* What harm could it do for me to try different treatments for my cancer? If there was another option available that made any sense, I probably would have considered it. At that time (1996), my prognosis for a success-ful outcome was slim to none. What did I have to lose?

Spoiler Alert

For your information, you might like to know that Kahlil Gibran also wrote the phrase, "Ask not what your country can do for you, but what you can do for your country," which is mistakenly credited to President John F. Kennedy. The actual phrase is from "The New Frontier," which Gibran had written thirty-six years earlier. His exact quote is, *"Are you a politician asking what your country can do for you or a zealous one asking what you can do for your country?"*

After reading Dr. Quillin's book and having decided to move forward with my nutritional approach (different diet and taking supplements) alongside the chemo and radiation, I had a follow-up appointment with my doctor. I recall specifically asking him, "What should I eat?" Diane was sitting in the doctor's office with me, pen and tablet in hand, and a blank page. The doctor informed us, "Eat whatever you want, but try to stay with a low-fat menu." This was not the answer I expected. I expected a list of items that I should not consume and one that I could eat that would benefit me in my fight against cancer.

Now there are two possible reasons the good doctor advised me as he did. One is that he was totally ignorant of nutrition (which unfortunately is true with most doctors). And two, he realized my dire situation and felt I would be dead within a year, so why restrict my diet? I suspect it was a combination of both. Diane and I left his office. Diane's tablet was blank just like it was when we arrived. It was now left to me to figure out what I should eat? No great diet or nutritional advice from the learned doctor!

In 1996 and even today, nutrition is not a major part of the education process for doctors. The medical community seems to be transfixed on *pills and procedures*; after all that is what they learn in college. If you have a chronic disease, the majority of doctors will give you a prescription (a pill) that will treat the symptoms but will not necessarily cure the disease. Is it in the doctor's best interest to cure you, or to give you some satisfaction and make it necessary for you to return to his office over and over? It has been proven that many chronic diseases (*diabetes, heart disease, high blood pressure, and obesity*) can be cured by diet alone! Fortunately, people are finding this out every day. Several doctors are going against the medical establishment and have started to inform the public of the great benefits of changing their diets to a whole food-plant based diet.

Go to YouTube on the Internet; in the search box type any one of the following names: Dr. Neil Bernard, Dr. Caldwell Esselstyn, Dr. Colon Campbell, Dr. John McDougall, Dr. Patrick Quillin or Dr. Dean Ormish. If you have a chronic disease or cancer, the videos that play for you will be an awakening! *Listen and learn.*

As evidence of what I'm saying about diet, let's look at my cholesterol in particular. Before my surgery, my combined cholesterol was three hundred sixty plus and it was like that for years. I was overweight and ate anything I wanted. After my lifestyle change and diet adjustments, my weight went down forty plus pounds and my combined cholesterol is always less than one hundred seventy. I would say that is quite an improvement without taking Lipitor or any other statins. The justification for prescribing Lipitor is that the reduction of the cholesterol will help improve your heart health. Well, losing a lot of weight will also improve your heart health. It will also drop your cholesterol numbers without exposing your body to statins, which are terrible for you.

Here is more evidence that diet works especially for heart patients. During the fall of 2015, I had the great fortune to rent a house to a wonderful couple, Theresa and Jim, from Cleveland, Ohio.

At the time I interviewed him, he was eighty-six years old. The reason I became interested in his story was because he was a vegan. When I gave them the keys to the rental house, he asked me if there were any vegan restaurants in the area. I told him where they were and I asked him why he was a vegan. He told me his story and it blew me away. I made a video of the interview so I could tell his story exactly as he told it to me.

At age sixty, Jim was having discomfort in his chest, on and off, for a year. At sixty-one, it was bad enough that he went to a cardiologist. A stress test was performed with no negative results but the doctor put Jim on medication for the next two years. The medications were changed periodically during those two years. The medications didn't help, and the pain was still there. Jim went to the Cleveland Clinic where it was decided he had a blocked artery. The doctor advised Jim to have an angioplasty procedure (stints were not available at this time).

This procedure was good for about six to seven years. When the pain returned, Jim went back to the cardiologist, who told him he had a "stable angina." Jim was given new medications. A couple of years later the pain was so severe Jim went back to the Cleveland Clinic. At this point in Jim's life, he was told he had five blocked arteries that could only be corrected with bypass surgery. He had the five bypass surgeries. It took him about three months to recover. At this time Jim was around seventy years old and was able to go back to playing golf, bowl and enjoy life again.

About a year later the chest pains came back. He returned to the clinic and was now advised he had three more blocked arteries. This time they inserted three stints. The pain returned within a year. Jim returned to find out he had another two blocked arteries and two more stints were inserted. This continued until Jim received a total of **seventeen stints**. The seventeenth and last stint was inserted in 2008. The pain returned with another blocked artery. He returned to the clinic. The personnel at the clinic told him they couldn't do anything else for him. Their advice was for him to change his lifestyle. They didn't tell him how to do that — just to change his lifestyle. Jim stated he was never told to change anything about the way he ate during the whole time all these procedures were taking place. Jim is Italian and eats accordingly … nothing healthy.

He ended up going to the dietician at the clinic who advised him to read, "Prevent and Reverse

Heart Disease" by Caldwell B. Esselstyn Jr. M.D. Jim did read the book and immediately and completely changed his lifestyle seven years ago. Jim now plays golf, bowls, goes to the gym and takes his wife dancing two nights a week. His pain has never returned!

All of Jim's procedures and the expense of the procedures could have possibly been avoided if Jim had been advised to read Dr. Esselstyn's book in the first place. Jim's heart disease was all diet related!

4

MY DOCTORS

I never questioned the advice of my doctors. When I was informed that I had pancreatic cancer, the doctors laid out the procedure that I was to follow in the weeks ahead. First, there would be the surgery followed by four weeks of mending. After my recuperation from the surgery, the plan included six weeks of chemotherapy in conjunction with twenty-eight days of radiation, all administered *simultaneously*. Instead of going to the oncologist's office for chemotherapy injections on a scheduled routine, I was fitted with a Porta-A-Catheter. The "Port-a-Cath" is a great devise that was surgically inserted just below my right side collarbone in the muscle tissue and just under the skin. The result was a round convex bump resembling a boil about one inch in diameter. Additionally, a plastic tube was inserted into a vein to allow the chemical (poison) to enter my blood stream. The idea was to fit me with a small bag of 5-FU (Fluorouracil) and a pump that would continuously infuse the chemical into the vein twenty-four hours a day, seven day a week, two weeks on and two weeks off. The pump and bag of 5-FU were worn around my waist and fit neatly under my shirt. The pump made a swish sound every four to five seconds, only noticeable at night when I was trying to go to sleep. This devise made me very mobile and I was able to travel without incident and continue working while I was being treated. The chemo and radiation did make me very tired at times.

I was in my primary doctor's office for a follow-up examination after the Port-a-Cath had been inserted by the doctor who had done my Whipple surgery. I asked my primary doctor (who really was an idiot — remember someone has to graduate at the bottom of their medical class and I'm convinced he was the one) for a "handicap" tag for my automobile since I was still working while I was taking the chemo and radiation. I was flying to meetings every week and walking through the Atlanta airport parking area, which was extremely difficult now that I easily got tired. He said OK and left the room. I sat there for fifteen plus minutes and he never came back. I left the room to begin looking for him. I bumped into him in a hallway. He was talking to another patient about golf. I interrupted him and asked about my handicap tag. He looked at me with a puzzled expression and the idiot asked me, "What is your handicap again?" My god, I was just with the dope twenty minutes earlier and he didn't know what my handicap was! I answered immediately "a twelve" (golfers will know the meaning of my reply). I'm not sure if he realized the humor in my answer but to make sure I received my tag I explained I was "his pancreatic cancer patient." He excused himself and immediately returned with a piece of paper which he handed to me. This episode proved to me I was nothing more than a faceless patient that was good only for a monthly billing for this particular doctor.

In Georgia, where I lived at this time and I'm sure it is the same in many states, you have to present your doctor's request for a handicap tag to the State Patrol in order to be issued the proper tag — one is temporary (thirty days) and one is for five years. I waited in line until my turn to approach the lady behind the counter. I gave her my document. She was very nice but explained to me that she couldn't give me a handicap tag since the doctor hadn't filled in the request form properly, only signed it! (I told you he was an idiot!) I explained to her what I had and showed her my chemo pump and bag and I also told her no one survives pancreatic cancer. She looked at me for a minute and then looked at the paper in front of her. She began to write on the handicap tag request form and then issued me a five-year handicap tag. She was a lot more optimistic than my doctors. I was happy.

Most people consider their personal doctor to be the very best there is or they go by the recommendation of a friend who says "my doctor is the best in the city; go see him about your problem." Since my experience, my feeling has always been that a doctor — any doctor — is the one who graduated last in his class until he convinces me otherwise. I'm not impressed just because he has a white coat and stethoscope. When you are talking to a doctor about your cancer treatment, you need to know how many cases of your particular type of cancer he has treated and how many he has cured — not how many have gone into remission. *"How many cases of my type of cancer have you cured?"* There is a great difference between "remission" and "cured." Surgery, chemo, and radiation can stop or eliminate a tumor and put you into remission. Just because the doctor tells you that you are in remission, it doesn't mean your cancer is gone or eliminated or you are cured! It just means the tumor is not there anymore. However, your cancer may still be active in your body. Remember, the tumor is the result of your cancer, not necessary the cancer itself. Changing your lifestyle as I did after I read Dr. Quillin's book and adopting a plant-based diet will certainly change the dynamics of the "tree in the woods" and hopefully your overall outcome. You have to understand, most doctors are compassionate and concerned about your well-being. The problem is they are not trained in alternate theories of treatment and are blind to anything that may offer a better outcome for your case. If a treatment isn't part of the major treatment structure offered by the current medical community, surgery, chemo, and radiation, the doctor isn't going to bring into the mix anything that opens him up to being sued. It is truly sad that we live in such a litigation-crazy society.

5

CANCER

Cancer is interesting. It has been with us as long as man has been alive. Cancer's history is sordid. There is a terrific book about cancer's history, "The Emperor of All Maladies," written by Siddhartha Mukherjee. I suggest you read it as well as all the other books I mention in this book. Cancer has been a real challenge to understand through the ages, even as it is today. With all the modern technology available to man, science still hasn't found the final solution to the cancer problem. There has been an on-going debate between the best way to prevent and cure cancer between the medical community and the groups that advocate a natural course to the prevention and cure of this devastating disease. We seem to be nibbling at the edges with minor results...

6

IRELAND

Diane and I were having dinner with two of our best friends, John and Debra Supple, one night in September 2015. John looked at his phone while we were waiting for our food to come and he asked, "Who wants to go to Ireland for a week for seven hundred ninety-nine dollars?" I immediately wanted to know how much was the airfare? John proceeded to tell us everything was included, even a car. Apparently, Groupon was having a special and the four of us were about to be the beneficiaries of this amazing deal. In the middle of December 2015, we ended up in Limerick, Ireland, at Adare Manor — a five-star hotel, golf club and manor house. The trip and accommodations were amazing. One night before having dinner in the manor house, we were asked to wait in the library prior to being seated. We were browsing the many magnificent books lining the multiple shelves waiting for our seats when Diane screamed, "Bob, look what I found!" She handed me a little five-by-seven inch, hard-bound, twenty-seven-page book titled "Cancer, Its Cause and Prevention," by Melville C. Keith, M.D., late professor in the Indiana Physio-Medical College, USA, published in 1905. The Indiana Physio-Medical College became extinct following its merger with the Indiana University School of Medicine in 1908. I quickly browsed the book before they called us for dinner. At dinner (which was spectacular, I might add … no meat for me), all I could think of was having that book. The next day, I went to the manager of the resort and told her I was working on my book about my experience with pancreatic cancer and would like to purchase that particular book for reference. She advised me that it wasn't for sale. She did offer to make color copies for me, which I gladly accepted. We were checking out the following day. Just before leaving, I received a message that the manager wished to speak to me. I visited with her on our way out, and to my surprise she had spoken to the owner of the property and he told her to give me the book. Again, I was happy.

This little book is amazing in the fact it documents the ongoing battle between natural cures and medical cures for cancer at that time. This battle has been going on well before the 20th century.

The following is from Dr. Keith's book, "Cancer, Its Cause and Prevention."

If we go to the medical "authorities" as to what is called "cancer" we shall find this following definition. It is taken from the "PRACTICES OF MEDICINE" by Robert Bartholow, M.A., M.D., LLD. He is, or was, "authority" among the allopath's, the "regulars" who dose out calomel after the practice of a quack named "Hohenheim", of the fifteen century. Bartholow was one of the men who lied about the native herbs of America. We are quoting from the sixth edition published by Appleton and Co., of New York, 1886.

Bartholow commences his article by saying "Etiology."

This word "Etiology" is made from the two Greek words "aitis-cause" and "Logos-word," which might be liberally translated by saying a word on the causes. Etiology is defined in Webster as being "that branch of medicine that treats of cause." So that when Bartholow writes "Etiology" we may suppose he is going to favor us with the causes. Bartholow will give us large words enough, but he is not writing for the heart-sick person who is afflicted with cancer. He is writing for the young medical priest who is just starting out in his career and these large words are needed in the business of gulling those who think they should have a knife stuck into them or who believe that some mineral or poison can do them some good in their bodies.

We should preach you a sermon on this hardness of heart which the medical priests have to acquire before they are allowed to "register" as "scientific" enough to deal out the worse then useless poisons but we do not have the time and postpone that part of our duty until later on. We are concerned with what this poison-dosing doctor may have to offer on the causes of "cancer." Here are his causes:

The points of election for the development of cancer in the intestinal canal, named in the order of their relative frequency, are the stomach, the rectum, the caecum, and the flexures of the colon. Of all the organs of the body, the stomach is most frequently the seat of cancer, more frequently than the uterus, which comes strictly next. As regards age, the majority of cases occur at fifty but the disease may appear at any time between forty-five and sixty. It is rare from thirty to forty. According to some authorities, cancer attacks the male sex by preference but careful investigation shows this view erroneous and that the two sexes are about equally divided. The well-to-do classes are said to be more liable to the disease than the poor and the obese, hardy feeders rather than the abstemious, but these are doubtful propositions.

*Predisposition and heredity play an important part in the causation of cancer; they are doubtless the most influential factors. The inherited tendency may not be traced sometimes when it exists because the behavior of the **cancer germ** skipping over one or more generations and appearing in subsequent ones. All other presumed moral and dietetic causes are rather fanciful.*

Here we have a leading doctor of the period stating **"dietetic causes are rather fanciful!"** Later in the book, Dr. Keith offers his causes of cancer, which are also incorrect but much closer to reality! He is surprisingly accurate by identifying a poor diet: eating pork, drinking alcohol, coffee, tea, gluttony, not keeping clean and smoking — correctly identifying nicotine as a definite cause of cancer.

You have to keep in mind, during this period in medical history the theory of germs was just accepted, leading most doctors to subscribe to the idea that cancer was caused by germs. Also during this time in medical history there existed allopathic doctors, which treated the symptom of a disease with chemicals or surgery, while homeopathic doctors treated the disease with the body's own functions or herbs. There were other forms of doctors as well: chiropractors, osteopaths and naturopathic doctors, to name a few.

Becoming a doctor at that time was nothing like it is today, thanks to the Flexner Report. In 1905, Abraham Flexner, a brilliant educator, was commissioned by the Carnegie Foundation to do an evaluation of all the medical schools in the U.S. and Canada. He compared them to John Hopkins. As a result of his efforts, almost fifty percent of the medical schools were forced to close. Those that didn't close were made to come up to the John Hopkins standard as far as admissions, teaching and hospital associations. The schools that adapted were the ones that were teaching surgery, radiation and using synthetic drugs. Those schools were given millions of dollars by the Carnegie Foundation with the help of John D. Rockefeller. With the advent of anesthesia, infection control and school certification, a new industry was born. Drug manufacturing exploded. The AMA quickly jumped on board supporting this new industrial medical model. The AMA declared anybody practicing medicine other than a doctor graduating from one of the accredited schools was a "QUACK." Advertising in the AMA Journal (JAMA) increased over five hundred percent in ten years. By the 1940s, the AMA had files on over three hundred thousand people they labeled as quacks. The AMA did do a lot of good for the general public by identifying many dangerous and lethal products during this time period. Unfortunately, they used a very broad brush to paint everybody as a quack even though there were several programs that were working at that time curing cancer using means other than surgery, chemotherapy and radiation. Instead of investigating these "alternate" cures, the AMA did everything they could to shut down the doctors or organizations that had proven results curing cancer.

Dr. Max Gerson and his Gerson Diet was one of the many victims of the AMA and the medical community in their battle against quacks. Gerson was the first major doctor to declare that smoking was dangerous. This declaration was especially upsetting to Dr. Morris Fishbein, editor of JAMA. The Phillip Morris Tobacco Company was the largest advertiser in the AMA's medical journal. Even though Dr. Gerson had documented evidence that his diet therapy cured cancer, Dr. Fishbein crushed him with his influence throughout the medical community. The AMA would not test Dr. Gerson's diet nor would they allow any of Dr. Gerson's papers to be published. At that time it was against the law to treat any cancer patient with any unaccepted therapy. The only accepted therapies were surgery, chemotherapy and radiation.

Because of many complaints, in 1953, the U.S. Senate enlisted Benedict Fitzgerald to investigate allegations of conspiracy and monopolistic practices on the part of orthodox medicine. Mr. Fitzpatrick's work uncovered enough information and proof that the AMA, JAMA (Journal of the American Medical Association) and at one time the president of the AMA and several national cancer organizations were guilty as charged.

"My investigation to date should convince this committee that a conspiracy does exist to stop the free flow and use of drugs in interstate commerce which allegedly has solid therapeutic value. Public and private funds have been thrown around like confetti at a country fair to close up and destroy clinics, hospitals, and scientific research laboratories which do not conform to the viewpoint of medical associations."

There were additional cures that Dr. Fishbein and the AMA tried to eliminate. Probably the most famous cancer cure was offered by Harry Hoxsey. This individual was a real character — a showman. He would perfectly fix the description of a "hustler" except he had a product that worked! The Hoxsey clinics were treating cancer patients in several states. He started in Illinois and came to the attention of the AMA. They wanted him to demonstrate his treatment to them. He did and it proved to be quite successful. Several of the AMA doctors wanted to buy his formula including Dr. Morris Fishbein. Hoxsey refused and went his way. The AMA swears this never happened. Hoxsey became a major target of the AMA and especially Dr. Fishbein. Over a twenty-five-year period, Hoxsey was arrested and challenged over and over. Finally Hoxsey sued the AMA and Dr. Fishbein. As a result, much to everyone's dismay, Hoxsey won the case. During the trial, Dr. Fishbein admitted that the Hoxsey treatment for external cancer worked (even though two federal courts had already found that his therapy worked)! He also had to admit that he, Dr. Fishbein, failed anatomy in medical school, became a journalist before he completed his internship, and had never treated a patient. After this fiasco and with a proven treatment for cancer, even the National Cancer Institute (NCI) refused to test the Hoxsey treatment for cancer. It was banned from use in the U.S., forcing the clinic to reopen in Mexico.

Another cancer treatment that never realized a real chance to be tested by the medical establishment was Dr. Ernest Krebs' work with Laetrile, commonly known as vitamin B-17. It was banned from the U.S. and labeled as quackery. However, Dr. Kanematsu Sugiura, a cancer researcher at Sloan-Kettering when he tested Laetrile, wrote a report and stated it was more effective in the control of cancer than any substance he had ever tested. The hospital demanded him to withdraw his findings. He would not. Sloan-Kettering later denied his findings. It was discovered that the people who were making the decisions concerning the information given to the public (board of directors and top management at Sloan-Kettering) were either invested in or worked for companies that made chemotherapy drugs, tobacco products and industrial chemicals. It certainly appears there was a massive conflict of interests involved in the results of an honored scientist's work and the interest of the general public. This incident with the suppression of the research on Laetrile led to the writing of the book, "The Cancer Industry," by Ralph W. Moss, former science writer at Sloan-Kettering.

There have been many more treatments that were never given a real chance at being tested and possibly approved by the government. Some may have worked or they may have really been quackery. We will never know. It appears that the AMA, FDA and the NCI are not interested in anything that treats cancer unless it is on their terms?

I am not endorsing any of these alternative approaches to cancer treatments. They are only included here so you can see that the AMA, NCI, FDA and other federal agencies are not your friends when it comes to cancer.

Just a side note ... in August 1987, the AMA was found guilty of "conspiracy" to destroy the chiropractic profession.

7

WHAT I FOUND OUT
ABOUT VITAMINS

We have dietary deficiencies that cause chronic diseases, and then we are treated by doctors who cram us full of prescription pills that only treat the symptoms of the disease and offer no real cure. We don't have a pharmaceutical deficiency, so why do we end up with a medicine cabinet full of different medicines?

There are 13 essential vitamins:

- A-Retinol

- B1-Thiamine

- B2-Riboflavin

- Niacin, B6

- Pantothenic Acid

- B12

- H-Biotin

- Folate

- C-Ascorbic Acid

- D

- E-Tecepherol

- K

- 8-10 amino acids

- 21-23 minerals

- 2 essential fats

Essential vitamins are organic compounds that are absolutely necessary to keep you alive. It is believed that we do not need massive amounts of vitamins. It is really unknown our actual need of all vitamins and minerals. Some have been identified because of deficiencies and serious illness that were the results of those deficiencies.

A government recommended daily amount (RDA) of vitamins has been made available to the public. It is one-size-fits-all, and in the past these types of guides were totally worthless. The FDA, which sets the RDA requirements, has not set the required amounts for the following:

Pantothenic acid (vitamin B5, which is vital to living a healthy life) and like all B complex vitamins it helps the body convert food to energy.

Biotin (sometimes referred to as vitamin H) is essential for the formation of fatty acids and blood sugar and aids in the metabolism of carbohydrates, fats and proteins.

Vitamin K is needed to help form coagulation of the blood for adults.

There is also not any set RDA for infants less than a year old. Doctor Suzanne Humphries, MD, has proposed that sudden infant death syndrome (SIDS) is caused by a vitamin C deficiency in infants.

The body makes four conditional essential vitamins, and sometime they need to be supplemented, as the body does not make enough. Most animals produce their own vitamin C. Only fruit bats, guinea pigs, primate monkeys and humans do not synthesize vitamin C. It has to be ingested.

Each vitamin performs a specific function in the body and they are critical to life itself. Without them the body stops living ... you die. We get vitamins from our food and or supplements. Fortunately we do not need them in large quantities.

Vitamins are either fat soluble or water soluble. Fat-soluble vitamins are stored in the body and only depleted when the body uses them. Water-soluble vitamins are not stored by the body, are continually depleted and need to be replaced. Most people don't realize they are taking supplements every day in their processed food that they purchase at the local grocery store. Pick up the cereal box in your cabinet and read the contents label. All grain products seem to have supplements added by the manufacturer, because all the healthy and good stuff originally in the grain has been removed during the processing of the product, leaving only empty calories. Adding vitamins to our food products goes back to January 1, 1942, when the Food and Drug Administration recommended that processed flour be fortified with iron, thiamine and niacin, because it was learned that as many as a quarter of the men enlisting in the Armed Forces during World War II were suffering from malnutrition. All grains were thoroughly milled at that time because milling allowed a longer shelf life of the product, thus allowing more profits for the company. Soon thereafter, pasta, corn meal, grits and white rice were to see the fortification of those products as well. The practice continues today.

8

MINERALS

Minerals are a necessary requirement by the body for good health. A body that lacks minerals can display physiological or physical abnormalities. When the minerals are added back to the diet, the conditions correct themselves without additional medications. Normally minerals come from the soil. Unfortunately, the soils in North America have become dematerialized (soil samples show a lack of necessary minerals because of over farming). When fertilizers are used, no minerals are added back into the soil — only growth agents for the product being grown.

There are ninety-two known minerals and elements. Research has not discovered every use of them in the body. Most of these minerals are not needed in large quantities. Only the top twenty-one minerals are identified. *The rest are present in trace amounts in the body and may play a key role in our health, but their role, as yet, is unknown. Could it be that some individuals lose the ability to absorb the essential vitamins and minerals and experience a clandestine deficiency? Could that deficiency be expressed by turning on cancer cells?*

9

A VERY LUCKY MAN

When I asked my doctors why I was still alive after five years, my medical professionals all told me, collectively and unanimously, it was without question that *I was lucky* (a new medical diagnoses). With that kind of information, I made sure I bought a lottery ticket every week. I didn't win anything.

10

"LUCKY AGAIN"

During 2001, Diane was having a lot of indigestion problems. Her doctor recommended that she have her gall bladder removed. Today the procedure is done by laparoscopy surgery. Generally it is outpatient surgery, unlike when my mother had her gall bladder removed in the 1950s. During the 1950s, gall bladder surgery was a major operation. After my mother's surgery, it took her a couple of weeks before she was able to leave the hospital. Diane went for her surgery in the morning, and that afternoon I picked her up at the doctor's office and took her home ... amazing.

During one of Diane's visits to the surgeon, she happened to tell him that I had had pancreatic cancer and a Whipple procedure. The surgeon told her I probably did not have pancreatic cancer and was misdiagnosed. "Nobody lives after a Whipple procedure. That's why I stopped performing them!" When I heard this, it made me mad. The next time Diane had an appointment with this guy, I made sure I took all my medical records and especially my pathology report with me so I could show him I, in fact, did have pancreatic cancer and a Whipple procedure. After he reviewed them, his only comment was, "*You are lucky.*" There it was again! That new medical term ... "*You are lucky.*" As I have always said, someone has to graduate last in his class. Perhaps the reason this guy's Whipple procedures were not successful wasn't the operation but the surgeon? Certainly makes one stop and think. Diane's operation was successful and she hasn't had any problems since. Perhaps this surgeon should stick to laparoscopy surgery!

In the beginning of my journey I tried to read everything that I could find on the subject of cancer and how to survive it. A lot of the books I read were junk. However, some of them really started to convince me that I had chosen the right path to follow with my diet and supplements. In addition to Dr. Quillin's book ("Beating Cancer with Nutrition"), I read "Cancer, Curing the Incurable," by Dr. William Donald Kelley, a dentist. The book is about the program he developed to cure himself of pancreatic cancer. It was very similar to Dr. Max Gerson's protocol that Dr. Gerson developed in the early 1930s.

Doctor Gerson was a very early proponent of better health through diet. He suffered from terrible migraine headaches and was able to halt them with an *elimination* diet. While treating a patient with his migraine diet, Dr. Gerson noticed the patient's skin tuberculosis was also cured, along with his migraines. This was extraordinary since tuberculosis was incurable at the time. Dr. Gerson's diet was picked up as a treatment for tuberculosis after that diet was put to a clinical trial test of four hundred fifty incurable skin tuberculosis patients. Four hundred forty-six of those patients completely recovered, resulting in a ninety-nine percent recovery rate and establishing Dr. Gerson's diet as the first cure for skin tuberculosis.

Dr. Gerson became close friends with Dr. Albert Schweitzer (Noble Prize winner) after Dr. Gerson cured Dr. Schweitzer's wife of lung tuberculosis with his diet when all conventional treatments at that time had failed. Dr. Schweitzer's type II diabetes was also cured by following Dr. Gerson's diet. This is what Dr. Albert Schweitzer had to say about Dr. Max Gerson.

"...I see in him one of the most eminent geniuses in the history of medicine. Many of his basic ideas have been adopted without having his name connected with them. Yet, he has achieved more than seemed possible under adverse conditions. He leaves a legacy which commands attention and which will assure him his due place. Those whom he has cured will now attest to the truth of his ideas."

Basically, Dr. Gerson's diet consists of a low-salt, low-fat, and high-carbohydrate diet plus oral administration of minerals and vitamins to supplement those vitamins missing in the diet. The diet also includes organic fresh fruit and vegetable juices and does not allow any meat, dairy, canned or bottled foods. Alcohol and tobacco of any kind are strictly forbidden. Similarly, Dr. Kelley's program incorporated much of the same. Dr. Kelley's approach also relied on Dr. John Beard's findings that he published in 1902 (more about Dr. John Beard later in the book). Dr. Kelley and Dr. Gerson were both dismissed by the established medical community in the U.S. as pure "quacks" even though both doctors were having very good results with cancer patients.

11

FOOD FOR LIFE

Some fifteen years later (I was still on my regimen), I was fortunate enough to learn about a *FOOD FOR LIFE* program that was being offered in Fort Myers, Florida. During my first meeting, I was discussing my cancer history with Kathy Reynaert, nutrition coordinator for the Fort Myers CHIP program, and Jean Struve, nutritionist for Lee Memorial Hospital. Both were working together conducting the class I was attending. Kathy's father had died from pancreatic cancer. They both asked me if I had read "The China Study" and if I had seen the video, "Forks over Knives." I told them I had not. Both insisted I read the book and see the video. I did ... thank God! Everyone reading this book needs to read "The China Study" and see "Forks over Knives."

After reading Dr. T. Colin Campbell's book, I now know why I survived my cancer. I was doing a lot of what Dr. Campbell explains in his well-documented study about cancer and how to prevent it. It was so simple. ***Animal protein feeds cancer!*** Eliminate animal protein in your diet and you starve cancer. I was doing the perfect follow-up to any standard cancer treatment and I didn't know it! I wasn't "lucky," which was the only explanation my doctors had for why I was alive.

I was doing what *every* cancer patient should do during and after their treatment ... eliminate animal protein from their diet! This program isn't just for a follow-up treatment. If a person follows a plant-based diet, they are potentially reducing their chances of turning on that renegade cancer-causing gene hiding in their body.

I had already stopped eating any meat from animals with a hoof per Dr. Patrick Quillin's book. I had already stopped all alcohol consumption.[5] I made sure no hydrogenated oils were eaten at any time, which meant that I never ate bread or rolls in a restaurant, potato chips or other snack foods. Fried foods were never eaten again. I took massive amounts of supplements including 6 grams of vitamin C daily.

---

5   Alcohol is the leading risk for disease and premature death in men and women between the ages of fifteen and forty-nine worldwide in 2016 accounting for nearly one in ten deaths. According to a study published by The Lancet.

.

There has been a lot of controversy about vitamin C and cancer. Dr. Linus Pauling, who was a world-renowned chemist and winner of two Nobel Prizes, did extensive research on this subject and concluded that vitamin C can prevent cancer. Dr. Pauling's theory has been challenged repeatedly by the medical community (more about vitamin C later in the book).

12

CHEMOTHERAPY

The history of chemotherapy is very interesting. When a test subject responded to a chemical injection of mustard gas and his tumor shrunk it was declared a success, even though the subject died shortly after the experiment. However, Doctor Sidney Farber was able to get folic acid antagonists to combat childhood leukemia in 1947. Because of his research and successes, Dr. Farber is regarded as the father of modern chemotherapy. It wasn't until the late '60s and early '70s that this form of cancer treatment was beginning to be accepted as a treatment for all cancers. Up until the 1960s, surgery and radiation were the primary accepted treatments. During this period, chemotherapy was still fighting for its place in the mix for cancer treatments. Today it is a process that most cancer doctors will recommend as a treatment in addition to surgery and radiation.

There are hundreds of different types of cancer. Cancers that respond well to chemotherapy are mostly the blood-related cancers: Hodgkin's disease, Leukemia, Lymphoma and testicular cancer. Several studies have shown that chemotherapy is effective when these types of cancers (blood-related cancers) are included in the study. When solid-tumor cancers are included, the studies show a very different result since these cancers do not respond very well to chemotherapy. The results of chemotherapy treatments are all over the charts. It is hard to say chemotherapy doesn't work, because sometimes it really does! I would say taking **all** cancer cases treated with chemotherapy, the results are minimal ... unfortunately.

I like to compare chemotherapy to the "transorbital lobotomy" that was developed in 1935 to treat mental illness. Dr. Walter Freeman, who in 1945 invented a simple way to perform a lobotomy (sometimes referred to as the "icepick lobotomy"), made it possible for thousands of these procedures to be performed even into the 1970s. This procedure was developed before there were antipsychotic medications. In the movie "One Flew over the Cuckoo's Nest," Randle Patrick McMurphy, a rambunctious but sane man, was confined to a mental institution. He was given a lo-botomy, which left him mute and feeble-minded. In reality the movie is very accurate. The effects of a lobotomy resulted in a third of the patients being helped, a third with no result or their con-dition made worse, and a third dying as a result of the procedure. I consider chemotherapy a total "body lobotomy." The only difference between the lobotomy statistics and the statistics for chemo-therapy is lobotomies statistics are much better.

13

ATHENS, GEORGIA

Diane and I went to Athens, Georgia, recently to a funeral service and to pay our respects to her high school sweetheart, who died of pancreatic cancer. The service was well-attended, as Mike Williams had a lot of lifelong friends and was well-respected in the community. I was sitting in the church thinking that he died of pancreatic cancer and I was told his doctors were treating him for acid reflux — how could this be possible? Poor Mike experienced the classic symptoms of pancreatic cancer but his doctors seemed to miss the obvious. He was experiencing upper stomach pain, which his doctors diagnosed as acid reflux. They diagnosed the acid reflux in August 2017. His pain continued to get worse. Nothing they gave him was working. One night in February, Mike was doubled up with so much pain his wife, Peggy Sue, took him to the emergency room at the local hospital. The doctors had to give him a shot to kill his pain so he could lie flat on the examining table. The emergency room doctors realized what he had was not acid reflux! On February 26, 2018, Mike was diagnosed with pancreatic cancer. On April 26, Mike passed away. He was given experimental drugs, chemotherapy, and not very much hope for a positive outcome.

How could his doctors have missed these obvious symptoms? It seems to be a common function for the doctors in Athens, Georgia, to misdiagnose pancreatic cancer. We had gone back four years earlier to attend the funeral of Diane's younger brother, Richard. He also died of pancreatic cancer. His doctors were treating him for fibromyalgia for a solid year and a half before he was diagnosed with pancreatic cancer. While we were in Athens for Mike's funeral, we stayed with Richard's wife, Sandy, who told me she had two friends who recently died of pancreatic cancer and both were misdiagnosed. What is wrong with the medical community in Athens, Georgia? I'm sure it isn't just those doctors who misdiagnose this terrible and deadly cancer. It is a hard cancer to detect, but there is a test available that can tell if there is cancer activity in the pancreas — the CA-19-9 blood test.

The CA 19-9 Radioimmunoassay (RIA) is a simple blood test that measures the level of tumor-associated antigens found in the blood. Antigens are substances that cause the immune system to make a specific immune response. CA 19-9 antigens are foreign substances released by pancreatic tumor cells.

It is important to note that not every patient with pancreatic cancer will have an elevated CA 19-9 level. In addition, some non-cancerous conditions can cause high CA 19-9 levels. For these reasons, the CA 19-9 test cannot be used as a diagnostic or screening test for pancreatic cancer even though 80% of the patients with pancreatic cancer will have elevated levels of CA-19-A.

What you just read is the reason this test isn't used when pancreatic cancer is suspected. I cannot believe that when a person presents a series of symptoms to a doctor, that doctor will continue treating the patient with their first diagnosis when the patient isn't responding! Anytime there is an upper stomach issue that isn't responding to treatment, I would suggest the CA-19-9 blood test just to make sure the pancreas isn't involved! My primary physician gave me two hepatitis C tests when I first went to him, knowing that that test was not accurate, and even telling me so when the first test came back negative. He never diagnosed my pancreatic cancer. He sent me to a gastroenterologist to see if he could figure out what my problem was.

While in the church, I had the pleasure of listening to Mike's brother-in-law, Bobby Poss, tell everyone how much he loved Mike and how he and Mike, over the years, would find themselves in rather interesting circumstances. Bobby reminded all of us he never called Mike by his first name — it was always *"brother-in-law."* Bobby began to tell us that he, brother-in-law and Bobby's father, Bob Poss, were all on a fishing trip when they passed a poster proclaiming that there was a tent revival in town that night. Brother-in-law studied the poster and said, "When we finish fishing tonight, I want to go to this revival."

Bob and Bobby agreed that it might be fun. When it was time, the three of them walked over to the large tent filled with a couple hundred people and took their seats. Bobby swore it must have been one hundred twenty degrees inside the tent, since the revival was taking place in the middle of July in Georgia. To further impress his point about the heat, he claimed a dog chased a cat through the tent, and both of them were walking! As the revival progressed, the preacher got to a point in his sermon that he asked people in the congregation who were having a problem to come forward, let the preacher touch them and then pray over them. Brother-in-law jumped up and grabbed Bob and Bobby, telling them, "I have to go down there to see that preacher." When the three were standing in front of the gentleman, who was just screaming about hellfire and damnation, he looked at brother-in-law and asked him, "What's yer problem, son?" Brother-in-law immediately said "my hearing..."

He was not able to complete his sentence and the preacher could not understand him completely because of all the screaming and yelling and waving of arms in the air. The preacher grabbed brother-in-law by the head, with his hands over his ears, and began to howler, shaking brother-in-law's head from side to side. He kept looking up towards the top of the tent. Within a minute or so, the preacher took his hands off brother-in-law's ears and pushed him back into Bob and Bobby's arms. The preacher looked straight into brother-in-law's eyes and yelled in his loudest voice, "Is yer hearing fixed?" Brother-in-law fired back at the preacher and proclaimed in his loudest voice, "I don't know; it isn't until next Wednesday."

The two preachers who were there to conduct Mike's service were visibly amused, as both were laughing out loud.

Bobby continued with the same fishing story.

The next day Bob, Bobby and brother-in-law were on the river in their boat fishing and noticed a group of people on the bank of the river gathered around the revival preacher from the night before, who was standing in the water. He was baptizing people. Bob, Bobby and brother-in-law decided to move a bit closer so they could hear what was going on. The revival preacher was asking a fellow who was in the water with him and who had had too much to drink the night of the tent revival, "Have you found Jesus?" The drunk didn't answer, and immediately the preacher dunked him in the water. After a short time under water, the preacher pulled the drunk out, looked him straight in the eye, and again shouted, "Have you found Jesus?" Again, there was no response from the drunk. And again the preacher proceeded to put the drunk under water, only this time it was twice as long as the first time. When the preacher pulled the drunk up, he shouted, "Have you found Jesus?" There was no answer, except the drunk was making gasping sounds. The preacher was getting very upset, so he put the drunk under water for a third time. He held him there much, much longer, and when he pulled him up, this time the drunk was coughing hard and spitting water everywhere. Again, the preacher screamed at the drunk, "Have you found Jesus?" The drunk, after he got his breath, asked the preacher, "Is this where he went in?"

At this point, the two preachers at Mike's service were holding their sides because they were laughing so hard.

It was a wonderful celebration of Mike's life! I was happy.

14

MY REGIMEN

At this point, I hope you have decided to change your lifestyle? I'm going to share with you exactly what I did after I was given the news that I had a terminal cancer. I would suggest you adapt this regimen and stick to it if you are being treated for cancer or as a follow-up after your cancer treatment. Remember, you have to be completely committed to a plant-based diet if any of this is going to work for you. There is no such thing as "a little pregnant" — you either are or are not. After reading several of the books I mentioned earlier, it was clear to me I needed to keep my nutritional needs satisfied. I had to eat even if the food tasted awful, which it did during chemo. I had to eat even if it hurt to swallow, which it did during chemo. I had to keep myself nourished – which I did!

I am not a doctor nor do I profess to have any cures or treatments for cancer. What is listed here is a regimen I developed for myself twenty-one years ago. It certainly has worked for me. It may sound strange to say, but the best thing that happened to me was getting cancer. Today, I am healthier and stronger than I was when I was diagnosed twenty-one years ago. I look at my friends as we all age together, and it is clear to me that I'm not aging as fast as they are. I am in better health than most of them. I have no complaints: I sleep at night; I have no acid indigestion, which I had every day and night prior to being diagnosed with pancreatic cancer; and all my plumbing works. In fact, at age seventy-five, everything works as it was designed to. I'm very happy to be alive.

If you elect to follow anything in this book, be sure and tell your doctor what you are doing and all the supplements you are taking.

1. Stop all consumption of any kind of alcohol.

2. Stop eating any meat that comes from an animal with a hoof.

3. Stop eating anything with hydrogenated oil in it. I avoid, as best I can, all **_hydrogenated oils_**. It seems that all food manufacturers use these cheap oils whenever they can. They are loaded with trans-fatty acids and are terrible for you.

Several manufacturers are now trying to change from this ingredient and are advertising on their packages "NO TRANS-FATTY ACIDS" i.e. Frito-Lay. These oils are in almost all baked and cereal (unless they are whole-grain) items you buy in a supermarket. Start reading labels and you will be amazed how much of this crap we eat on a daily basis. Another of the big offenders is margarine. Margarine is generally hydrogenated oil. Read the labels on the packaged food you purchase. If you can't pronounce what is on the label, don't eat it — better yet, don't buy it!

As of May 2018 the World Health Organization (WHO) has announced a plan to eliminate all trans fat from our food, worldwide. They say it is responsible for over 500,000 deaths a year attributed to heart disease.

4. Do not eat or drink any milk products. If you want something to drink or put on cereal, use almond milk or something of that nature, plant-based.

5. Eliminate all fried foods. The problem with fried foods is the oil used to cook them. Before it's heated, frying oil is made up mostly of triglyceride molecules. But when it's used to fry foods at high temperatures — about 160 C to 170

C — thermal changes occur in the oil. It becomes hydrolyzed. Hydrogen molecules from steam react with oil chemicals, making new chemicals, subject to oxidation, which causes chemicals in the oil to react with oxygen molecules in the air. The result is an unhealthy chemistry. Some of the chemistry's components simply disappear into the air as a gas, but others — such as polymers and free fatty acids — remain and change the oil's chemical composition. To make matters worse, oil is absorbed more readily by food, filling it with even more chemicals. Need I say anymore?

6. Do not drink carbonated beverages such as Coke, Pepsi, etc. Do not drink diet drinks with artificial sweeteners under any circumstances. Do yourself a favor and watch the documentary video on YouTube, "Sweet Misery."

7. Eliminate caffeine in your diet (I have done this with the exception of two cups of coffee in the morning. I drink the two cups of coffee, no more, for the laxative effect, which works like clockwork). Caffeine is generally an additive in all soft drinks.

- Avoid sugars as much as possible. Stevia is a natural sweetener, if necessary.

In a study at UCLA in 2010, researchers found tumor cells that fed on both glucose and fructose used the sugars in two different ways. Both sugars fed cancer cells but the fructose caused pancreatic cancer cells to proliferate!!! The sugar industry states "sugar is sugar"...[6]

---

6   Anthony Heaney of UCLA's Jons son Cancer Center

15

WHAT I DO EAT AND DRINK

1. Fresh vegetables

2. Fresh fruits

3. Water (I drink water with all my meals — no tea, no soda, nothing except water).

4. One hundred percent whole grain either in the form of bread or cereals. Read the label and if it says Multi-grain, generally, it isn't whole grain. It will have processed flour as a component.

5. I graze daily eating nuts or some fruits.

6. Periodically I will allow myself a small piece of fresh fish or even a smaller piece of baked white meat chicken (three to four ounces every two to three weeks, no more)!

7. Smoothies with fruit, almond milk, and *vegetable* protein powder (no whey protein pow-

der as it is made from milk and has casein in it, which is animal protein, which cancer feeds on). Sometimes I also add chopped-up kale to the shake. You can buy it in bulk in the vegetable section of any grocery store and take it home, freeze it, and use it over several weeks. Works great with frozen bananas to make the smoothies cold and thick.

16

SUPPLEMENTS

I take a lot of vitamins.

The vitamins listed here are taken on a daily basis. Also, it is important to take capsules instead of tablets when available. Capsules, generally liquid or powder, are adsorbed earlier into the system and do not travel through the digestive track as a mini compacted brick as do most multi-vitamins. *Under no circumstances take these vitamins on an empty stomach ... unless you really want to feel bad!* I have added a brief explanation to some of the items you may not be familiar with. After reading about them, you will understand why I take them as part of my regimen.

Vitamins, Minerals and One Unknown (CoQ10)

1. Vitamin C, I take 2 (1-gram capsules) every time I eat. I take at least 6 grams of vitamin C a day.

Do not start out taking 6 grams a day. You have to work up to that much. Start with 1 gram 2 times a day and after a few weeks start adding an additional gram to your regimen, which is what I did.

When learning about this fantastic vitamin, you need to read about Dr. Frederick R. Klenner, M.D. Dr. Klenner did amazing, documented work with high doses of vitamin C in the 1940s. He successfully cured sixty cases of polio with vitamin C alone. He even presented his work to the Annual Session of the American Medical Association on June 10, 1949, in Atlantic City, New Jersey:

"It might be interesting to learn how poliomyelitis was treated in Reidsville, N.C., during the 1948 epidemic. In the past seven years, virus infections have been treated and cured in a period of seventy-two hours by the employment of massive, frequent injections of ascorbic acid, or vitamin C. I believe that if vitamin C in these massive doses — six thousand to twenty thousand mg in a twenty-four hour period — is given to these patients with poliomyelitis none will be paralyzed and there will be no further maiming or epidemics of poliomyelitis."

None of the doctors in attendance nor did the AMA have any interest in Dr. Klenner's cases. In later writings, Dr. Klenner described a five-year-old girl that he treated for polio in 1951. She had been paralyzed in both her lower legs for over four days. She was in pain. Four consulting physicians confirmed the diagnosis as polio. Massive vitamin C injections were given. The only other treatment was massage. After four days, the child was again moving her legs. The child was discharged from the hospital. She was given one gram of oral vitamin C every two hours for seven days. After nineteen days of treatment, the child was cured, with no long-term, devastating or crippling result for the remainder of the girl's life.

Klenner would say, "When proper amounts are used, it will destroy all virus organisms. Don't expect control of a virus with one hundred to four hundred mg of vitamin C."

2. Pancreatic Enzyme, (Creon 12-prescription only) I take one capsule three times a day and one at bedtime. You can get pancreatic enzyme at any vitamin store. Mine is by prescription required by my surgeon after my operation and will be something I take the rest of my life. Since I only have two-thirds of my pancreas still functioning, the pancreatic enzyme helps me break down proteins I ingest when I eat. I'm not sure if his prescribing the pancreatic enzyme for me had anything to do with the pancreatic enzyme

theory that was incorporated by Dr. Kelley and Dr. Nicholas Gonzales in their protocols. The theory follows:

A key concept underlying the original use of pancreatic enzymes for cancer treatment is what is known as the trophoblastic theory of cancer. When a human egg is fertilized by sperm, the early cell divisions produce a small ball of cells, which give rise to the blastocyst (preimplantation embryo). The blastocyst possesses a surrounding layer of cells known as the trophectoderm, which is made of individual cells called trophoblasts. Responsible for protecting the developing blastocyst and for mediating its attachment to the wall of the uterus, trophoblasts create the placenta. During the process of attaching the blastocyst to the uterine wall, trophoblasts express invasive qualities similar to those found in cancer cells. Trophoblasts, however, cease their invasive activity once the placenta is in place and functioning and then differentiate into other cell types.

When Scottish embryologist Dr. John Beard first observed the invasive activity of trophoblasts in 1902, he speculated on the similarities between these cells and cancer cells. In addition, he observed that trophoblast invasiveness begins to decline at about the same time that the pancreas in the developing fetus begins to function. He also theorized that maternal pancreatic enzymes might play a role in containing trophoblastic in-

vasiveness in the uterus. These considerations led to his proposal that cancer cells, like trophoblasts, arise from primordial germ cells. Dr. Beard also thought that some of these primordial cells — carrying latent capacities for invading tissues — could escape and spread throughout the body of the developing fetus. Because he thought it possible that pancreatic enzymes modulated the degree of trophoblastic invasiveness in the uterus, he suggested that these same enzymes play a role in either limiting or eliminating cancerous cells elsewhere in the body. Dr. Beard worked before the advent of molecular biology and human genetics. Although unable to experimentally establish that pancreatic enzymes had anticancer effects, he published papers and a book about his theory between 1902 and 1911. Other scientists of the time raised significant objections to the trophoblastic theory of cancer, and it was never broadly accepted.

As Dr. Beard had before him, Dr. Kelley also asserted that trophoblasts and cancer cells have a common origin in primordial germ cells. Dr. Kelley maintained, furthermore, that cancer was initiated when primordial germ cells migrated to a point in the body already weakened by toxic exposure and nervous system imbalance. At these presumably compromised sites, the germ cells met no opposition from the immune system and initiated an aggressive invasion of normal tissue, creating malignancy. Dr. Kelley's treatment approach was based on the belief that primordial germ cells are the single cause of all cancers, no matter where they occur, and that pancreatic enzymes are able to suppress or destroy cancers.

3. Vitamin E 400 I.U.

4. Selenium (most of the soil in the U.S. is depleted of this important mineral)

5. Garlic

6. Beta-Carotene 15 mg

7. B-Complex including B12

8. Calcium plus Magnesium

9. Flaxseed oil capsule or freshly ground flax seeds in my morning oatmeal.

10. A Men's Multi-Vitamin (Women should take a Women's Multi)

11. CoQ10 300mg, this is probably the best antioxidant available today. A substance found in most tissues in the body, and in many foods. It can also be made in the laboratory. It is used by the body to produce energy for cells and is a very powerful antioxidant. CoQ10 is a ubiquinone; that means it is found in every cell in the body. As we get older, the body tends to make less of it. The medical community doesn't know how to

classify this substance. They are not sure if it is a vitamin or a mineral — who cares if it helps. I have taken this religiously for twenty-one years. Some very well-known cosmetic companies advertise it as an important ingredient in some of their skin revitalizers.

12. IP6 is something of an unknown that is being looked at by some cancer researchers. It has proven to be effective in reducing liver tumors. I have taken it for over ten years. It comes from brown rice. Here is some info on this substance:

Inositol hexaphosphate (IP6) is a naturally occurring polyphosphorylated carbohydrate that is present in substantial amounts in almost all plant and mammalian cells. It was recently recognized to possess multiple biological functions. A striking anticancer effect of IP6 was demonstrated in different experimental models. Inositol is also a natural constituent possessing moderate anticancer activity. The most consistent and best anticancer results were obtained from the combination of IP6 plus inositol. In addition to reducing cell proliferation, IP6 increases differentiation of malignant cells, often resulting in a reversion to normal phenotype. Exogenously administered IP6 is rapidly taken into the cells and dephosphorylated to lower-phosphate inositol phosphates, which further interfere with signal transduction pathways and cell cycle arrest. Enhanced immunity and antioxidant properties can also contribute to tumor cell destruction. However, the molecular mechanisms underlying this anticancer action are not fully understood. Because it is abundantly present in regular diet, efficiently absorbed from the gastrointestinal tract, and safe, IP6 holds great promise in our strategies for the prevention and treatment of cancer. IP6 plus inositol enhances the anticancer effect of conventional chemotherapy, controls cancer metastases, and improves the quality of life, as shown in a pilot clinical trial. The data strongly argue for the use of IP6 plus inositol in our strategies for cancer prevention and treatment.

13. Alpha-lipoic acid is something I have been taking for over fifteen years and here is why: If its essential role in health is any indication, alpha-lipoic acid may very well join the ranks of vitamins C and E as part of your first line of defense against free radicals. Discovered in 1951, it serves as a coenzyme in the Krebs cycle and in the production of cellular energy. In the late 1980s, researchers realized that alpha-lipoic acid had been overlooked as a powerful antioxidant.

Over the past few years, the pace of research on lipoic acid has increased dramatically. Several years ago, Lester Packer, PhD, of the University of California, Berkeley, published a lengthy review article on alpha-lipoic acid in Free Radical Biology & Medicine (1995;19:227-

50). In April 1996, he presented a short review of it in the same journal (FRBM;20:625-6).

Several qualities distinguish alpha-lipoic acid from other antioxidants, and Packer has described it at various times as the "universal," "ideal," and "metabolic" antioxidant. It neutralizes free radicals in both the fatty and watery regions of cells, in contrast to vitamin C (which is water soluble) and vitamin E (which is fat soluble).

The body routinely converts some alpha-lipoic acid to dihydrolipoic acid, which appears to be an even more powerful antioxidant. Both forms of lipoic acid quench peroxynitrite radicals, an especially dangerous type consisting of both oxygen and nitrogen, according to a paper in FEBS Letters (Whiteman M, et al., FEBS Letters, 1996; 379:74-6). Peroxynitrite radicals play a role in the development of atherosclerosis, lung disease, chronic inflammation, and neurological disorders.

Alpha-lipoic acid also plays an important role in the synergism of antioxidants, what Packer prefers to call the body's "antioxidant network." It directly recycles and extends the metabolic lifespans of vitamin C, glutathione, and coenzyme Q10, and it indirectly renews vitamin E.

In Germany, alpha-lipoic acid is an approved medical treatment for peripheral neuropathy, a common complication of diabetes. It speeds the removal of glucose from the bloodstream, at least partly by enhancing insulin function, and it reduces insulin resistance, an underpinning of many cases of coronary heart disease and obesity. The therapeutic dose for lipoic acid is six hundred mg/day. In the United States, it is sold as a dietary supplement, usually as fifty mg tablets. (The richest food source of alpha-lipoic acid is red meat, which I don't eat.)

"From a therapeutic viewpoint, few natural antioxidants are ideal," Packer recently explained in Free Radical Biology & Medicine. "An ideal therapeutic antioxidant would fulfill several criteria. These include absorption from the diet, conversion in cells and tissues into usable form, a variety of antioxidant actions (including interactions with other antioxidants) in both membrane and aqueous phases, and low toxicity."

"Alpha-lipoic acid...is unique among natural antioxidants in its ability to fulfill all of these requirements," he continued, "making it a potentially highly effective therapeutic agent in a number of conditions in which oxidative damage has been implicated."[7]

These are the supplements that I have taken in addition to my diet. There are a lot of doctors who say it isn't necessary to take supplements. "You get all your nutrients and vitamins from your food"... Really?

---

7   The Nutrition Reporter

How can you get all your nutritional needs from food that has been produced in fields stripped of natural nutrients and grown with only chemical: nitrogen, phosphorus and potassium? According to the Nutrition Security Institute (www.nutritionsecurity.org), U.S. soil is eroding ten times faster than it can be replenished. Researchers who compiled reports from around the world conclude that U.S. agricultural soil has been depleted of eighty-five percent of its minerals and vitamins during the last one hundred years.[8]

Despite my doctor's advice about diet, I decided to venture into supplementation on my own. I had never taken a vitamin or mineral in my life. Would I kill myself with an overdose of anything higher than the recommended daily allowance (RDA), which is the gold standard of the U.S. government? Having decided I would start to self-medicate myself with vitamins and minerals, I wanted to speak to Dr. Quillin myself.

At that time, Dr. Quillin was the Director of Nutrition, Cancer Treatment Center of America in Chicago, Illinois. (Cancer Treatment Centers of American was the only cancer hospital at that time that offered the three standard cancer treatments: surgery, radiation, chemotherapy and **nutrition** as a treatment for cancer.) I was

---

8   Health Freedom Advocate

interested in the nutrition part of their protocol! I wanted this meeting with Dr. Quillin before I started my chemo and radiation treatments because I intended to take these supplements during my treatments.

On my appointment day, Dr. Quillin was called out of his office for an emergency. I was directed to meet with his assistant, at that time, Dr. Kim Dalzell (at the time we met Dr. Dalzell wasn't a doctor). She and I talked and I presented her a list of the vitamins I had prescribed for myself based on what was in Dr. Quillin's book. I wasn't sure if I was taking the correct amount. I wanted to know if I was going to kill myself from a vitamin overdose. Much to my surprise, Dr. Dalzell dramatically increased everything I was taking and also added CoQ10 (coenzyme Q10). Since she recommended it, I have taken it every day for the last twenty-one years. Dr. Dalzell was nice, informative and offered me a lot of hope and encouragement. *After our meeting, I was positive and filled with hope. I left knowing I was going to beat my pancreatic cancer! I was happy.*

Dr. Dalzell has a very informative website www.challengecancer.com that outlines the best healing plant and natural medicine strategies for sixteen kinds of cancer based on cell type and common genetic mutations associated with those cancers.

A lot of the vitamins I take now, I have acquired along the way over the last twenty-one years and were not a part of our original discussion. They are ones that I have added. Most are antioxidants and designed to help strengthen my immune system.

17

WHAT THE DOCTORS TOLD ME

After my treatments and the fact that I didn't die, my doctors were amazed. When I reached the two-year milestone, they really began to take notice. Some of them were interested in what I was doing, especially my oncologist. I saw him more than the rest of my doctors, so he was more familiar with my routine. He gave credit it as part of the reason for my survival. He even hired a full-time nutritionist to consult with his patients.

Five years into my survival, I asked each doctor — surgeon, oncologist and radiologist — if they would take credit for my survival. Each one said no. They did tell me "not to stop whatever I was doing." I have not stopped, and I'm still here twenty-one years later, watching everything I eat.

"Stop Feeding Your Cancer," written a few years ago (2014) by Dr. John Kelly, MB, an Irish general practitioner, is worth mentioning. Dr. Kelly became aware of Dr. Colin Campbell's book "The China Study," in which Dr. Campbell made a compelling case for the fact that animal protein feeds cancer. Dr. Kelly was amazed there wasn't much excitement within the medical community about Dr. Campbell's research.

Dr. Kelly was so convinced by Dr. Campbell's research that he decided to introduce the idea of a plant-based diet to his cancer patients. Those patients that seriously followed the regimen remained alive while the others that went on with their normal diets all died from their cancer. These results are not a scientific study, only the results of a very concerned doctor for his cancer patients' well-being. Dr. Kelly is convinced the dramatic results are directly attributed to the plant-based diet!

I read everything I could about pancreatic cancer and cancer in general. Most of it was not supportive of the outcome I wanted. That didn't discourage me. You need to do the same thing I did: *read, read, and read some more.* I have given you the names of several books to read and several YouTube videos to review.

Remember the things I did were part of several larger programs developed by well-respected doctors or scientists at the time. All had successes and were quickly dismissed by the medical community and their results never were seriously tested. My approach can be looked at as a smorgasbord solution. There are elements I have taken from Dr. Gerson, Dr. Quillin, Dr. Linus Pauling, Dr. William Kelley and Dr. T. Colin Campbell. Remember, my regimen was done in conjunction with the standard cancer treatments offered to me at the time my cancer was diagnosed.

If I had to do it all over again, I'm sure I would do the same thing I did originally. There have been a lot of advancements in cancer treatment since I was diagnosed. I would be a lot more cautious today than I was twenty-one years ago. I would not say yes to anything my doctor offered without a lot of explanation and statistics to back up whatever he was telling me.

After I started my regimen, people couldn't believe how positive I had become during my treatments. When I went to my oncologist's office to get my bag of poison, everybody there looked so miserable. I was there always smiling because I knew I was doing something in addition to my chemo and radiation treatments that would support the outcome I wanted. I was in this battle with my doctors and very positive about winning my war with pancreatic cancer — which I did. And that makes me very happy!

My advice to everyone with cancer or who has already been treated for their cancer is to consider doing the following to make sure your cancer stays in remission or doesn't spread or return:

1. Start a plant-based diet immediately. (Thank you, Dr. Campbell)

2. Read all the books mentioned in this book.

3. Watch YouTube videos by the doctors mentioned in this book.

4. Visit any website suggested in this book.

5. Changing your lifestyle is hard — stick with it and don't give up. It works.

6. Take vitamin supplements.

7. Be positive — keep smiling.

8. Don't always believe everything your doctor says. Do your own research!

9. Keep smiling — there is always hope for survival!

10. And most importantly, "Look both ways when you cross the street."

MAKE A COMMENT

If you would like to make a comment about this book, you can do so at:

robertbeatspc@gmail.com

I'm not a doctor and I do not give medical advice, so please do not ask me for any. However, I would suggest you get a vitamin and nutrition profile from any laboratory that provides this type of blood analysis. The test will help you know what vitamins and nutrient deficiencies you have and will help guide you in designing your own regimen.

Another important book to read is "Cancer Secrets" by Jonathan Stegall, MD. Dr. Stegall is an integrative oncologist who incorporates alternative cancer therapies with standard chemotherapy.

Made in the USA
Monee, IL
15 August 2023